Y0-ELU-769

Sex, Guilt & Forgiveness

JOSH McDOWELL

POCKET GUIDES™
Tyndale House Publishers, Inc.
Wheaton, Illinois

Pocket Guide is a trademark of Tyndale House Publishers, Inc.

Library of Congress Catalog Card Number 89-52193
ISBN 0-8423-5908-7
Copyright © 1990 by Josh McDowell
All rights reserved
Printed in the United States of America

95 94 93 92 91 90
 8   7   6   5   4   3   2   1

CONTENTS

Acknowledgments

Thanks to:

Don Smedley for his assistance in writing and editing;

John Harris for scrutinizing the manuscript;

Becky Bellis for extensive research on sexual abuse and date rape;

Dave and Neta Jackson for preparing the manuscript for publication;

Jan Frank for permitting the inclusion of a personal interview with her on sexual abuse.

Additional thanks to the following people for their assistance in developing the content of chapter 5:

Dan B. Allender, Associate Director, Institute of Biblical Counseling, Morrison, Colo.;

Becky Bellis, writer and editor, Salem, Ohio;

Cheryl Biddle, Lee Gsellman, and Kaye Malyuk, Akron Pregnancy Services,

5

Akron, Ohio;

Barry R. Burkhart, Ph.D., Professor of Psychology at Auburn University, Auburn, Ala.;

Kevin M. Huggins, M. Div., M.A., Associate Pastor and Director of the Youth Division, The Chapel, Akron, Ohio;

The Minirth-Meier Clinic, Richardson, Tex.;

Norm Wakefield, Ed.D., Shared Life Ministries, Phoenix, Ariz.;

Peg Zeigler, Director of Rape Crisis Center, Grady Memorial Hospital, Auburn, Ala.

Sex and Guilt

"I hold a respectable job, am active in my community, have a lovely wife and three children. My job takes me out of town occasionally and that's when it happened. I consistently had illicit sexual affairs while away from home and my wife has just learned of them. I feel so guilty and ashamed. For a fleeting foray of pleasure, I have risked reputation, position, career, income, family, marriage, and the goodwill and trust of many friends. How can I live with myself? The guilt and the shame is overwhelming. Can you help me?"

—Unfaithful Husband

"I could not break free from the bondage of having sex with Curt. It ruled my life. How cheap and dirty I had become in my own eyes.

"Sex gave me the loneliest thrills I had ever experienced. It handed me fear as a gift and shame to wear as a garment. It blinded

*my eyes to false love and gave me a jagged
tear in my heart that even now, seven years
later, is still healing."*

—Still Healing Single

*"I had sex with my boyfriend thinking I owed
it to him. . . . Later when I learned I was
pregnant he blew up and said I should get an
abortion—that it was all my fault. So, to
save my parents heartache and to keep Matt,
I had an abortion. Now Matt has left me.
How can God love me after all I have done?
I'm just so confused. Can God really love and
forgive me?"*

—Confused Teenager

THE BONDING FACTOR OF SEX

I'm convinced after receiving letters like
these and facilitating countless counseling
sessions that sex is one of the most powerful elements in our lives. Sex was created
with a powerful bonding factor to bring two
committed, married people together in a
powerful way. It was never designed to
lead to "the loneliest thrills I have ever
experienced."

The power of sex can either bond our
relationships together or blow us apart
emotionally—often with guilt, shame, or
intense emptiness. Sex can and will become a positive bonding factor in our lives
when we follow the clear instructions from
the creator of sex—God. In part, God created sex to be within marriage to end

human loneliness. "It is not good that man should be alone" (Genesis 2:18). But isn't it ironic that the very thing God has given us to end human aloneness proves so often to cause it?

FORGIVENESS: ANTIDOTE TO GUILT

Yet, I am here to say that with all the broken hearts, guilt, stored-up grudges, resentment, and bitterness, there is a solution. The product of sexual misuse and abuse that is tearing apart relationships, destroying lives, and dividing families can to a great degree be resolved when people *know they're forgiven and then become channels of forgiveness to other people.*

When Billy Graham spoke in Honolulu, a group of twenty respected psychologists were sent to listen to his sermons and write up their criticism for the newspapers. They all agreed on one thing in their reports: When Dr. Graham called on people to repent and receive God's forgiveness, his advice was psychologically sound.

Probably the most frequently asked question that I get as I speak to young people around the country is "Can God really love and forgive me?" The question almost always relates to sex and usually to premarital sex. Young people just don't believe that God can forgive them. They think that their sin is too great or that somehow because it's a sexual sin, they'll never be able to feel forgiven.

That's just the opposite of everything that God has said in the Bible.

DAVID'S STORY

First, in God's eyes, sex is not a sin! Not one verse in the Bible says that sex is in any way wrong or dirty. In fact, it's quite the opposite. Every reference to sex in the Bible either declares or presumes that it is beautiful.

So where did the popular notion come from that God disapproves of sex? Well, it probably arose from a misreading of the verses in the Bible that say the *misuse* or *abuse* of sex is sin. And you have to have something good before it can be misused or abused.

One of the best known examples of what happens when a person doesn't follow God's original design is the ancient Israeli King David. His affair with Bathsheba, another man's wife, has been the favorite focus of Hollywood movie-makers. But what we usually fail to see portrayed on the screen is David's inner struggle with what he'd done. He described how it felt this way: "When I kept silent, my bones wasted away through my groaning all day long. For day and night your hand was heavy upon me; my strength was sapped as in the heat of summer" (Psalm 32:3-4).

Have you ever felt that way? David couldn't eat; he struggled all day; he was feeling the heat. He felt God convicting him to deal with what he'd done. That's the way God designed us to operate. The best way to deal with these feelings is head-on, as David eventually did.

Actually, before David was finished, his sin also included murder as he attempted to cover up his adultery. But God still called King David a man after his own heart. That's right—the Bible describes David as a man after God's own heart. Let's consider the sequence of events that led to his sin and recovery.

One night, during a stroll on his rooftop, David got into trouble. He became the first recorded biblical Peeping Tom, a voyeur. He peeked over the side of his roof and saw Bathsheba, the wife of one of his soldiers, taking a bath.

It was no sin for David to have accidentally run across Bathsheba bathing. But David did more than notice her; he gazed at her, he chose to continue spying on her. David looked, and *then* he got hooked. He sent for Bathsheba and brought her up to his palace, had intercourse with her, and got her pregnant.

Immediately after hearing that Bathsheba was pregnant, David attempted a cover-up. He brought her husband, Uriah, back from war for a little R and R. If Uriah would sleep with Bathsheba, it would appear that he had impregnated her. But Uriah was so distraught about the plight of his comrades back in battle that he didn't go home. David resorted to having Uriah murdered in battle so that he could take Bathsheba as his own wife "legitimately."

As with most things of this sort, David probably didn't fool very many people. The palace gossip line probably had the full story. And finally God sent the prophet Nathan to confront David about his sin. Nathan told David a story that was so powerful that it drove David to his knees. Here it is:

> There were two men in a certain town, one rich and the other poor. The rich man had a very large number of sheep and cattle, but the poor man had nothing except one little ewe lamb he had bought. He raised it, and it grew up with him and his children. It shared his food, drank from his cup, and even slept in his arms. It was like a daughter to him.
>
> Now a traveler came to the rich man, but the rich man refrained from taking one of his own sheep or cattle to prepare a meal for the traveler who had come to him. Instead, he took the ewe lamb that belonged to the poor man and prepared it for the one who had come to him (2 Samuel 12:1-4).

When David heard this, he became very angry. You see, he didn't realize Nathan was speaking allegorically. He thought Nathan was reporting an actual event that had occurred in his kingdom and wanted David to render a sentence against the unjust rich man. So David said:

> "As Surely as the LORD lives, the man who did this deserves to die! He must pay for

that lamb four times over, because he did such a thing and had no pity."

Then Nathan said to David, "You are the man!" (2 Samuel 12:5-7).

To David's credit, he didn't deny it. When confronted with his sin he acknowledged it.

David learned that whenever you break a moral law, your first sin is against God. So if you've had sex with someone to whom you are not married, you have not only wronged that person, you've wronged God. That's the first thing David learned.

At this point it's important to realize that David was called "a man after God's own heart" after he committed the sins against Bathsheba and her husband, not merely before. David *completely* acknowledged his sin, and God forgave him . . . *completely*. So the first step in getting rid of the guilt and hurt in your life and in gaining God's forgiveness is to own what you have done, acknowledging that you have really blown it. Whenever you believe that God can't forgive you, just remember David and read Psalms 51 and 32 very carefully.

CALL A SPADE A SPADE

Have you ever messed things up so badly that all you can think of is the fantasy of turning back time—"If only it were this morning," "If only it were the beginning of the summer and I could start over."

If you feel that way about a sexual sin you've been involved in, then I've got some good news for you. When the Bible talks about how we've really messed up, it uses the word *sin*—and God is in the business of forgiving sin!

Sin is the biblical word for having royally messed up. Thought of that way, it's no wonder the Bible says, "For all have sinned" (Romans 3:23). Certainly that's true! We've all messed up, we've all sinned—if not in one way, then in another.

No one likes to admit they've failed. We can easily blame others, or our circumstances, for our misuse of sex, for wrong decisions, for other kinds of failures. Blaming others is as old as Adam and Eve, as new as the next reported scam. Adam blamed Eve for giving him the forbidden fruit—as though he had no choice. Eve blamed the serpent for deceiving her—as though she didn't understand what was happening. Likewise, many of us are tempted to say, "Yes, I disobeyed God when it comes to sex. But I loved her [or him]! But I was vulnerable! But I had needs!"

All of that may have been true. But for God, the only thing that counts is , "God, I have sinned"—period! Sin is our own fault.

God knew what was happening in David's life. And God knows what's happening in your life. He knows everything about us. The Bible is clear that ". . . all things are open and laid bare to the eyes of

14

Him with whom we have to do" (Hebrews 4:13, NASB). At first that may seem intimidating—we can't hide anything from him—but when we understand that God's love for us is based on his knowledge of us, it can be comforting. Finally, finally someone *really* understands us.

Even more exciting than the thought that God really knows us is the fact that He really wants to help us. And that's what the Bible is all about. It's the story of how God cares so much for us that He wants to help us when we've messed up. And He's really the only One who can make it just as if "it were this morning," or just as if "it were the beginning of the summer." The process is called *forgiveness*.

The next chapter offers some steps that will help you bring God's forgiveness into focus.

Escaping the Guilt Trip

The director of a mental institution in Knoxville, Tennessee, once said that 50 percent of the patients could go home if they only knew and believed that they were forgiven. But how does one experience forgiveness—and so escape the guilt trip?

CONFESSION: GOOD FOR THE SOUL

The Bible says that for us to experience forgiveness, we must do three things. As we saw in chapter 1, the first step is our unqualified admission that we have failed.

After we admit that we have sinned, the second step is to confess our sins to God. Saint John explained: "If we confess our sins, he [God] is faithful and just and will forgive us our sins and purify us from all unrighteousness" (1 John 1:9).

The word *confess,* as used in this Bible verse, means "to say the same thing." In other words, to agree with God—to agree that we have sinned and that Jesus Christ died for our sins.

Maybe that's not hard for you to do, but frequently we are interested in justifying what we have done. We just can't admit that we've messed up. Sometimes this is because we are insecure, but occasionally we haven't yet seen the wrongness of our choices. Other times we don't want to give up our sin; we'd rather continue in it. But when God says, "If we confess . . ." it is also an admonishment by God *not* to do it again and a desire on our part to stop sinning.

Now, I know what's happening: your mind may be spinning with reasons you shouldn't *have* to confess your sin. So let's look at some of the common excuses before we go any further.

1. *"It was so long ago that I've almost forgotten about it."* Right, almost but not quite. God has something better for you. He wants it completely dealt with so that future events won't trigger a flood of thoughts that could lead to a round of paralyzing guilt.
2. *"But I don't think what I did was wrong; I don't feel guilty."* Flying through life by your feelings can lead to a crash. Not that feelings are unimportant. We need to pay attention to them. But they must be interpreted by more reliable information, an objective standard—in other words, what God says.

3. *"It might offend the person I was involved with if I bring this up."* Your primary offense was against God and that needs to be dealt with.

Confession is not only healthy for the spirit, it is also healthy for the soul. We're not telling God anything he doesn't already know! But through confession we enter into dialogue with Him so that He can begin the process of restoring us.

RECEIVING FORGIVENESS
John said: "If we confess our sins, he [God] is faithful and just and will forgive us our sins and purify us from all unrighteousness" (1 John 1:9). His instruction for how we can experience forgiveness is really in two parts:

1. We are to confess our sin, and when we do . . .
2. God will forgive and purify or cleanse us.

The final step in experiencing God's forgiveness has to do with the second half of John's advice. Not only does God want us to acknowledge our sin, He wants us to acknowledge (accept) His forgiveness of our sin. Why is that important?

In some cases, it may personalize or complete our process of confession. After all, some of us have trouble accepting forgiveness because deep down we don't really think we need it or possibly don't want it because we know our action is wrong but don't want to stop doing it.

Suppose you met an old prospector in the middle of the desert and said, "I sure am thirsty; can I have some water?"

"Sure thing, partner," answers the old prospector. "There's my canteen. Help yourself."

But if you didn't take him up on his offer and swallow a drink, you would not only miss the benefits of the water but you'd raise doubts about the credibility of your "confession" of thirst. This is because the nature of real thirst *compels* one to take advantage of water. You've got to have it. You've got to take it in and make it yours if it is offered.

Christ's death on the cross is the basis for our forgiveness. This is very clear in the Bible: ". . . we have been made holy through the sacrifice of the body of Jesus Christ once for all" (Hebrews 10:10). When He died on the cross 2,000 years ago, He died for every sin you ever committed— past, present, and future. So, as in the story of the prospector, the "water" of His forgiveness is there.

When we sin, we create a barrier between us and a perfect, holy God; the "thirst" is there on our part. But what happens if we don't acknowledge our need? David says, "If I had cherished sin in my heart, the Lord would not have listened" (Psalm 66:18). He's saying that if he hadn't acknowledged or forsaken his sin—if he had chosen to hide it in his heart—he couldn't have enjoyed the benefits of the forgiveness; the Lord wouldn't have heard him when he prayed.

Through confession we agree with God that our sin was wrong, we acknowledge it (as David did in Psalms 32 and 51 concerning his sin with Bathsheba), and then we can experience God's forgiveness. It is not so much that you feel different, although you very well may. But after confession, you realize that there no longer is that wall that you have erected between you and God.

You see, confession is not for God's benefit; He already knows what we've done. But the Lord requires confession of sin for our benefit, so that we can continually have, know, and experience a clean life through His love and forgiveness. This is the case even in—especially in—the area of sexual sin.

ALL-INCLUSIVE FORGIVENESS
Jesus died on the cross to take away God's punishment for our sins once and for all. Saint John built on that foundation when he wrote, "If we confess our sins, he is faithful and just and will forgive us our sins and purify us from all unrighteousness" (1 John 1:9). God didn't say all our unrighteousness *except* for sexual sins. Rather he said *all* unrighteousness

Why Sex Sins Are So Serious

God forgives sexual sins completely. From that perspective they are no worse than any other sin. But the practical consequences personally and socially are deeply damaging. Jack W. Hayford, the senior pastor of The Church on the Way in Van Nuys, California, offers the following explanations.

1. Sexual sins stain the deepest part of our identity. Our sexuality is foundational to who we are.
2. Sexual activity awakens our deepest passions, exposing us where we are most vulnerable emotionally.
3. In spite of the *fact* of God's equal forgiveness, sexual sins are the hardest

including sexual sins. To review: Which sins did that sacrifice cover? Everything but our misuse and abuse of sex? No. It covered them *all*. An infinite God can wipe the slate clean forever, for all time.

Not only that, but God also gives us a new life in Christ. After we accept His offer of forgiveness, we are no longer the persons we once were. Saint Paul pointed out:

When you were dead in your sins . . . God made you alive with Christ. He forgave us *all* our sins, having canceled the written code, with its regulations, that was against us and that stood opposed to us; he took it area for people to believe in God's forgiveness.

4. Marriage is the foundation for the deepest human relationship. Sexual sins compromise that foundation.

5. Sexual sins risk begetting unsupported human beings, a social phenomenon that has led many to the scandal of abortion.

6. Sexual sin increases the potential for disease.

7. Sexual sin breaks trust with the church community of interdependent relationships. The social fabric unravels if those relationships aren't dependable. It's not a private matter.

Adapted from "Why Sex Sins Are Worse Than Others" by Jack W. Hayford, *Charisma & Christian Life*, October 1989, pp. 68-74.

away, nailing it to the cross (Colossians 2:13-14, italics mine).

The death of Christ serves as a basis for our forgiveness; it gives us a new life; and, in addition, we now have someone who stands before God on our behalf at all times, namely Jesus. He always testifies that since we are now forgiven, we will always remain forgiven—no matter what. Even if we sin after we trust Jesus as Savior, we can still be forgiven. That's right! Saint John told us: "My dear children, I write this to you so that you will not sin. But if anybody does sin, we have one

who speaks to the Father in our defense—
Jesus Christ, the Righteous One. He is the
atoning sacrifice for our sins, and not only
for ours but also for the sins of the whole
world" (1 John 2:1-2).

A CLEAN RECORD

Right after I moved to Julian, California, a
beautiful little town up in the mountains
northeast of San Diego, I bought a diesel
Volkswagen Rabbit. It turned out to be a
dud on those mountain roads, so I had a
turbo charger put on—and convinced my
wife it made the car "safer."

The same day I picked up my modified
Rabbit, I had to go to Ramona, our closest
"city." On the way there's a long straightaway through the mountains. A motorcy-
clist was ahead of me, not going too fast, so
I decided to pass and pulled out. Well, he
figured he wasn't going to let some Rabbit
pass him and he stepped on the gas. There
I was with a new turbo charger, and I
thought to myself, *I might as well test it!* So
I floored it, and it really worked. I passed
that motorcycle doing eighty-five miles per
hour before the straightaway ended.

Two curves later, the biggest red lights
I've ever seen flashed in my rearview mir-
ror. A California highway patrolman pulled
me and the cyclist over and ticketed both of
us. I deserved that ticket. I had broken the
law and had no excuse.

But when I went to the courthouse in

Ramona to pay the ticket, the clerk said, "You don't need to pay this if you take a three-hour driver's safety class. Also, it will be removed from your record." So I did. When the class was over, I went back to Ramona with the little slip signed by the driving instructor. I gave it to the clerk, who said as she took it, "Your record is wiped clean."

After I was back in the car, it hit me: My record was clean. It was just as if the clock had been turned back to the morning and I had been given another chance. It was a powerful reminder of what Jesus Christ did on the cross with my sins. He wiped the record clean. He canceled my debt and made it possible for me to be reconciled to God.

So, you see, Christ's death serves as the *basis* for our forgiveness for all our past mess-ups, for all our present ones, and even for all our future sins. His death covered it all. But how do we experience this forgiveness for ourselves? Maybe you accept that God forgives all kinds of other sins, but sexual sins seem different to you. What happens when we feel so distant from God that we can't imagine ever getting back into His good graces? What can we do when we just plain feel guilty?

RELEASE FROM GUILT
David said in Psalm 32, "I acknowledged my sin to you and did not cover up my

iniquity. I said, 'I will confess my transgressions to the LORD'—and you forgave the guilt of my sin." Did you catch that? He dealt with your *guilt*.

Not just the sin is forgiven, but the guilt as well!

How complete is this forgiveness? One of the most significant verses on the extent of forgiveness tells us that "as far as the east is from the west, so far has he removed our transgressions [or sins] from us" (Psalm 103:12). Maybe you wonder why the Lord didn't say He would put your sins as far away as the north is from the south. Well, if the north and south had been used, one could have measured the distance between the poles. But not so with east and west. There is no east pole or west pole. If you start going east, you can go east for an eternity, and it's the same with west. The point is that you can't measure it. The distance has no boundaries; it's infinite.

That's how complete Christ's death on the cross is for your sins. Your record is wiped clean through the blood of Christ.

In the letter to the Hebrews God gives this promise:

"Their sins and lawless acts I will remember no more." And where these have been forgiven, there is no longer any [need for a] sacrifice for sin (Hebrews 10:17-18).

So often we don't realize the significance of Christ's death on the cross and how it relates to us. If only each of us could grasp the good news of forgiveness! The good news, the Gospel, is that Jesus didn't come to save righteous people. He came to save sinners! Those who have blown it. He isn't interested in our proving to Him how good we are. His message is forgiveness! Accepting the fact that we are sinners— that you and I sin—doesn't mean that we should wallow in our unworthiness. God wants to lift you up and set you free!

FORGIVING YOURSELF

Often we manage the first three steps quite well—call our behavior sin, confess it to God, and receive His forgiveness—and then we get stuck. We can't seem to forgive ourselves.

Forgiving ourselves can be the hardest thing of all. Somehow we think that we have to go out and do penance. One person said, "I understand what Jesus did for me, and I accept that. But I still feel like I need to do something to be able to forgive myself."

It can be one thing to know you are forgiven by God and another thing entirely to cleanse your conscience of the guilt that sin produced. We know that God has forgiven us; however, for some reason we seem to have a better memory for our sin than God does in situations like this. It seems that we have higher requirements for forgiveness than God does.

In order to free your mind and emotions

from the guilt that sin produces, you must not only acknowledge God's forgiveness but also forgive yourself. To do so, you must realize that God has no prerequisites before you can know you are forgiven, and that He desires no penance on your part. He loves *you*.

NO MORE GUILT TRIPS!

Let me illustrate. Early in my Christian life I would confess sins to God, acknowledge His forgiveness, then get down on myself for what I had done. Soon I was off on a huge guilt trip. Even though I knew God had forgiven me, I felt that I now had to prove I was worthy of that forgiveness. I thought I had to earn the right to forgive myself. I thought I could not make any mistakes in order to minister in Jesus' name. Isn't it interesting that we can be harder on ourselves than God is?

Well, some time ago, something happened to me that showed me clearly that the real issue in forgiving myself was not how many times or how badly I blew it. The real issue was how I responded to God when I *did* sin.

One day I was in a restaurant and I hurt someone deeply by saying something I should never have said. It was sin on my part. On the way home I realized the impact of my uncalled for, "off-the-wall" remark. Immediately I confessed my sin to God. I also realized I needed to return to the restaurant and confess my sin to the one I had hurt.

So I turned around, found this brother, and said, "What I said was wrong and I know I hurt you. I've confessed it to God, and I've come back to ask your forgiveness. Will you forgive me?"

To my amazement he said, "No. I won't forgive you. Someone in your position shouldn't have said that." After further discussion he still refused to forgive me.

I went home frustrated and confused. Soon I was off on another of my guilt trips, asking myself, "How could you have said that? How can anyone in Christian work hurt a brother like that? How can God use you now?" My self-chastisement almost sounded like a new song about the misery of personal guilt, "Oh, woe is me."

Do you see what I was doing? I was making forgiveness from a brother the prerequisite for being able to forgive myself. I was letting someone else's response control my life and relationship with God.

Then God started working on me. "Just a minute, Josh, you're not handling this right. You can respond in one of two ways: You can wallow around in guilt, focus on your failings—or you can realize that Jesus died for this situation. You have confessed it to God and to the one you hurt; so get on with your life!"

After wrestling awhile with the alternatives, I confessed the whole thing to God once more and then added, "And Father, I forgive myself, too." I determined to do all that I could from then on to heal the relationship with my wounded brother, but not to allow his response to impair my assurance of God's forgiveness for me.

As time went on I repeatedly went out of my way to express love to him. Finally, our relationship was healed, and reconciliation and forgiveness took place. In fact, the relationship is now better than it ever was before. This wouldn't have happened if I hadn't taken God at His word—that He does offer forgiveness—and then, based upon God's forgiveness, forgiven myself.

WHEN YOU REFUSE TO FORGIVE YOURSELF

One of the things that grieves God the most is for someone to reject or "cheapen" His grace. When we refuse to forgive ourselves, we are actually throwing God's loving grace, His unmerited favor, right back in His face. By not forgiving ourselves we are implying that Jesus Christ's death on the cross was not sufficient for all our sins. We are saying, "God, I'm a better judge of what and who can be forgiven than You are." Confession is agreeing with God not only about the wrong done, but also about what He did in forgiving the sin.

There is a freedom that comes with forgiving yourself. The following letter from Amy tells of the joy that can be yours through forgiveness:

Dear Josh,

What you said hit me hard. I never understood that I had to forgive myself. This week I have been let out of the cage that I made for myself. The cage was not forgiving myself. And boy, because I did not forgive myself, it affected my relationship with everyone, especially my boyfriend. I could love him unconditionally, but I couldn't let him love me unconditionally. Even though he forgave me for the things I did before becoming a Christian—you name them, I did them—I could not forgive myself. But since our talk I have forgiven myself, and in one day I have grown greatly. I wish you could understand my definition of my growth. It is just awesome!

Thank you for showing me that I can forgive myself because of Christ.

Sometimes, refusing to forgive ourselves is a form of pride. We think we should be beyond sin, so we refuse to accept ourselves as we really are—fallible human beings who are capable of blowing it, not just once, but again and again. The real issue in forgiving ourselves, however, is not in how many times or how badly we blow it. The real issue is how you and I deal with it when we do sin.

So forgive yourself. God does. And He loves you, too.

Forgiving
the Other Person

In Hawaii recently, a very sharply dressed man and his wife sat down near me. We struck up a conversation, and I inquired about his work. He explained that he was a consultant to corporations in the areas of personnel development and problems.

When I asked what problem he encountered most, he immediately replied, "Conflict."

Since I was preparing a series of talks on conflict resolution, I immediately asked, "What is the number-one way you have found to resolve conflict?"

Without batting an eye he responded, "Forgiveness." He said the greatest difficulty he faces is challenging people to give up their bitterness and to give and receive forgiveness.

This man clearly understood the importance of forgiveness.

WHY FORGIVE?

The Bible doesn't mince words when it comes to forgiving. We are *commanded* to forgive. Jesus told His disciples, "When you stand praying, if you hold anything against anyone, forgive him, so that your Father in heaven may forgive you your sins" (Mark 11:25). And again right after the Lord's Prayer, Jesus said, "If you forgive men when they sin against you, your heavenly Father will also forgive you. But if you do not forgive men their sins, your Father will not forgive your sins" (Matthew 6:14-15).

This seems to say that our own forgiveness is based on whether we forgive others, not on Christ's death on our behalf. But that would contradict the rest of Christ's teachings. Instead, I believe Jesus is saying that if we refuse to forgive someone who has wronged us, God will know our own confession of sins to Him is less than genuine—that we haven't fully received (or understood) the forgiveness He has freely made available. Our lack of forgiveness toward others is a clear signal to God that our confession of sin to Him was insincere.

There's another reason to forgive. Lewis Smedes, in his insightful book *Forgive and Forget* (Harper and Row, 1984) writes:

> Forgiveness is the only way to be fair to yourself. . . . Suppose you never forgive,

suppose you feel the hurt each time your memory lights on the people who did you wrong. And suppose you have the compulsion to think of them [or your hurt] constantly. *You have become a prisoner of your past pain.* . . . The only way to heal the pain that will not heal itself is to forgive the person who hurt you. Forgiving heals your memory as you change your memory's vision.

ROADBLOCKS TO FORGIVENESS

Let's face it. Knowing we *should* forgive and actually being able to forgive can be two different things. There are often roadblocks within ourselves or in the relationship that hinder us from forgiving.

- *Insecurity.* If we feel insecure in the relationship, we are going to look for every opportunity to build ourselves up in our own eyes and the eyes of others. Maintaining a position as "the injured party" can give a false sense of righteousness and status.
- *Holding a grudge.* In Ephesians 4:30-32 Saint Paul instructed us not to harbor bitterness, yet we all know we can take a kind of pleasure in such resentment. Some people are motivated by bitterness for a lifetime. It is possible to relish harboring a "right" to resentment. Some of the most infamous events in history were perpetrated because of a grudge.

35

- *Fear.* When you forgive someone, you make yourself vulnerable. If you've been burned or hurt before, unforgiveness builds a barrier around you; you may be afraid to let down that barrier and allow the relationship to come close, for fear of being hurt again.
- *Self-pity.* Sometimes our whole identity is built around self-pity. "I've been hurt more than anyone, poor me!" We find it hard to let go of our hurts; what will we talk about? If I'm not "poor, wounded me," who will I be? Even though the Bible assures us that God works all things (even the bad things) together for our good (Romans 8:28), we say in effect, "God, this area cannot work together for good, and You are powerless to do anything about it."
- *Plain old anger.* Your feelings are too new, too strong. How dare she or he do that to you! You want to hold on to your anger so the other person realizes the full effect of his or her dastardly deed.
- *Failing to forget.* Some people say they forgive, but they don't forget. Henry Ward Beecher explained that the phrase "I can forgive, but I can't forget" is only another way of saying, "I can't forgive." Forgetting doesn't mean that you can't recall the situation. Rather, it means that you're no longer controlled by the hurt or the desire to get even.
- *Pride.* Pride says, "I don't need to forgive and be reconciled because I don't need

this person. I'll just avoid the person; I can do without the relationship."

- *Judgment.* We decide that the person doesn't deserve to be forgiven. The hurt was too great; the person wouldn't change anyway. Forgiveness would be wasted on such a person. The offender needs to be punished, not forgiven! (Yet we don't ask ourselves: Do we deserve God's forgiveness?)
- *Revenge.* Sometimes our ability to forgive is smothered by a desire for revenge. We want to see the person who hurt us fail in an important project or relationship. We want him or her to suffer like we have suffered so they will feel sorry for what they did to us. We choose not to believe that God said, "Vengeance is Mine, I will repay" (Hebrews 10:30, NASB); we ignore Paul's instruction, "Do not repay anyone evil for evil" (Romans 12:17).
- *Lack of strength.* After a deep hurt, we simply may feel we're not emotionally strong enough to say sincerely, "I forgive you."

BURN NO BRIDGES

Given these hindrances to forgiveness, I still encourage you to engrave this phrase across the billboard of your mind: "When I refuse to forgive, I am burning a bridge that I will someday need to cross." No matter who you are, and more often than you can imagine, you are going to need forgiveness from someone else.

Who are you and I supposed to forgive? You must forgive anyone who has hurt you, abused you, or offended you. Maybe you carry bitter feelings toward a parent because of incest, divorce, abuse, or alcoholism. Maybe you still steam about how your first boyfriend took advantage of you. Maybe you've been involved in an affair that hurt you as well as your spouse.

No matter how bad a situation, God can use it for your good.

Does this mean it was a good situation? Absolutely not.

Can God redeem it? Yes.

Forgiveness changes the conditions under which we experience life. We live daily in the reality of God's forgiveness. He loves us. We are accepted by Him—not because we are perfect or deserve it or never make mistakes, but because He forgives us completely and wants us to be one with Him.

Corrie ten Boom experienced this need to forgive. Corrie and her sister, Betsy, were prisoners in Ravensbruk, one of the Nazi concentration "death" camps. Betsy died in the camp from ill treatment, but not before giving Corrie a vision that forgiveness is stronger than hate. After her liberation from the prison camp, not only did Corrie begin to share this newfound message of forgiveness, but she actually went back to Germany to *be* a messenger of forgiveness to the nation that had so abused her and her sister.

In Munich one Sunday, she was preaching her message of forgiveness. Afterward, one of the people standing in line to greet her was, of all people, a former guard who had tortured her sister. Not recognizing her, he thrust out his hand. "How grateful I am for your message, Fraulein," he said. "To think that, as you say, He [Jesus] has washed my sins away!"

Corrie was frozen. She immediately had recognized the man, his face so etched in her memory she could never forget it. She remembered how she was forced to take showers with other women, naked, while this beast looked on leering and mocking. She recalled the inhuman treatment of her sister whom she so loved. She couldn't forgive this man. She just could not!

But as the bitterness boiled inside her, she realized, as she already knew, that Jesus had died for this man, too. "Lord Jesus," she prayed silently to herself, "I cannot forgive him. Help me! Give me your forgiveness!"

Suddenly she felt a warmth come into her body, flowing through her to this man. She slowly took his hand, and into her heart sprang a love for her enemy that nearly overwhelmed her. And so her message of forgiveness continued on, a message so strong that even hate, humiliation and death could not conquer it.

FORGIVENESS IS NOT . . .

Often it is easier to understand what something is by seeing what it is not. I believe this applies to understanding forgiveness.

- *Forgiveness is not a feeling.* It is an act of the will. There have been times when I didn't feel like forgiving and had to do it by faith. Yet I can't remember a single instance of forgiving by faith when the feelings didn't come afterward.
- *Forgiveness is not pretending the situation never happened.* So often people just go on with life and act as though there never was a problem. Lots of families do this; when there is a conflict, everyone withdraws until it just kind of "blows over." But denying the problem doesn't end it; it just puts the problem on "simmer." If this is the way you are dealing with a situation, don't be surprised when it comes back in full steam.
- *Forgiveness is not condoning wrong.* Sometimes we fear that forgiveness will be misunderstood as being "soft on sin." Forgiveness helps us resolve the personal hurt, but doesn't mean we condone a wrong action. Jesus showed us how when He forgave the woman who had just been caught in adultery and said, "Go, and don't sin anymore."
- *Forgiveness doesn't mean there won't be consequences.* If you have been sexually abused and forgive the offender, that does not mean that you shouldn't report

the offense and insist that the person get professional treatment. If you are a woman and pregnancy results, it is still appropriate to expect the offender to shoulder the responsibility for supporting the child. This is not punishment but *restitution*. You can forgive the offender, but that person still has to deal with the law and the consequences of his or her action.

- *Forgiveness does not mean that the person you forgive is going to change*. Forgiveness can't be conditional: "If you promise never to do it again, I'll forgive you." Being forgiven often gives a person the courage and will to act differently. But your forgiveness should not be based on the person's future actions. Whether an offender gets help and truly changes may determine whether or not you can trust the person, but it need not be a condition for forgiveness.

- *Finally, forgiveness cannot insulate you against future hurts*. But if you can forgive now, you will be better able to deal with the conflict and hurts to come. And if you deal with hurts and resentments along the way, you keep them from festering and growing into much larger problems down the road.

WHAT FORGIVENESS IS
- *Forgiveness is an expression of God's love that takes the initiative*. Have you ever

41

thought, "Why should I forgive her? She hasn't even said she's sorry!" God's love, however, compels us to take the first step. In the Bible, Saint John wrote, "This is love: not that we loved God, but that he loved us and sent His Son as an atoning sacrifice for our sins" (1 John 4:10). If God had waited for us to repent and ask His forgiveness before reaching out to us, we would still be lost. But He took the first step—paying the death penalty for our sins—and then invited us to receive His pardon.

I, too, have a story of forgiveness; it involves my father. For years I hated him; to me he was the town drunk. I was often embarrassed to bring my friends over, afraid they would see him. So on occasion, when he was drunk, I would tie him up in the barn out of sight. I would put a rope around his neck, pull his head over the top board of a stall, and then tie the rope around his feet. That way, if he struggled to get loose, he would choke himself.

Well, shortly after I became a Christian, God began to give me a love for my father, a love that I had never had before. Soon I was able to look my father in the eyes and say, "Dad, I love you, and I forgive you." After some of the things that I had done and said to him, it really shook him up. And within a short time, I had one of the greatest privileges in my life—leading my father to Christ.

Finally I had realized that I had not been born to my parents by chance; God had handpicked them for me. God used my parents and the experiences of my childhood to make me who I am today, to form my character, to bring me to Himself. I needed to forgive my parents and be free of the resentments that kept me a prisoner of my own pain.

Usually changes take place gradually, but the life of my father changed right before my eyes. He touched whiskey only once after that. He brought it to his lips and put it down. He didn't need it anymore. Forgiveness changes lives; it is powerful.

Our society says, "You have rights. Demand your rights!" But God has called us to forgive those who tread upon our rights. This includes everything from insults to criticism to rejection to being sexually used and abused. Is this hard? Of course! In our own strength it is nearly impossible. But as Lewis Smedes writes, again in *Forgive and Forget,* "The linkage between feeling forgiven and the power to forgive is the key to everything else."

GENUINE RECONCILIATION
As we've seen, in most cases the objective of forgiveness is reconciliation. However, if you have been the victim of sexual abuse (see chapter 5), the idea of reconciliation with the person who violated you may seem utterly abhorrent.

In many regards, your intuition is right; you should stay away from that person until he or she has dealt with and been healed from the sinful behavior. Biblical reconciliation must not include putting you back into a dangerous position. Sometimes we are called to face danger or endure suffering, but that is not a reconciled situation.

On the other hand, a common reaction of those who have been abused is an inability to relate freely to anyone, even their trustworthy friends. Reconciliation in this regard means being able to relate to people normally and freely again.

But beyond this, if you were a victim of sexual abuse in the home where you grew up, you may have mixed feelings toward the offender. Maybe it was your father, uncle, brother, or mother. You may love the person and long for reconciliation—provided the past can be dealt with and your safety secured. This is where true forgiveness can lead to genuine reconciliation.

Breaking Free from the Past

You can't turn back the clock. That's the bad news. But the good news is that God is in the restoring business. He has given you a clean heart through His forgiveness. Now the question remains, How do you make a clean break from the past? How do you make a new start?

A CHANGE IN CONDUCT

A change in conduct should always follow a change in conviction. If not, the change in conviction wasn't really a change at all; it was only a nice idea.

The Bible tells us you can "Produce fruit in keeping with repentance" (Matthew 3:8). The word *repentance* means to change your mind. Thus, when we repent, we have a change of heart; we turn from one opinion to another. In the area of sexual sin, to repent means to change our mind from approving or justifying our past sexual behavior to following God's way of purity and respect.

Repentance means that by conscious decision, energized by God, we turn from our ways to God's ways. After we call our previous behavior sin, confess it, acknowledge God's forgiveness, and forgive ourselves, it's time to act differently. True repentance is *always* accompanied by action, the "fruits of repentance."

Let me offer you an illustration. Suppose you are a single woman. You and your boyfriend have had sex two or three times. Finally, God's conviction reaches you, and you know it's wrong. But you know the man well, and you know that he's not going to want to stop having sex. You confess to God, you acknowledge God's forgiveness, and you forgive yourself. Now, in keeping with your repentance, and with God's help, you will break off the relationship. You know you've got to do it, or you're going to slip back into your old behavior.

END IMMORAL RELATIONSHIPS
In most cases, when you do become physically involved, it is necessary to break up. Once you've had intercourse, it's hard to go back to holding hands! It's not quite the same.

Usually, you need to make the decision to break off the relationship *without* discussing it with the other person. Why? Because it's really your decision. *You're* accountable for your life. But if you submit the decision to your girlfriend or boyfriend for discussion, you have taken the first step of surrendering the whole decision.

Before you go to your friend, decide that you are going to break it off. You are not asking him or her for an opinion or for permission; it's not a request. Make the decision before God that the relationship is already over. Then your purpose in talking is to announce and explain your decision. It's not up for negotiation. That's fruit in line with repentance. In other words, your actions are a visible expression of your change of mind.

It doesn't mean that God might not bring you back together again. But once you've been involved physically, especially when sexual intercourse has taken place, most people need a break—a physical, emotional, and mental break—from the other person.

Maybe fruit in line with repentance for you is deciding not to go to "those" kind of parties anymore. Maybe it means resolving not to lie down on the couch with your girlfriend or boyfriend. Maybe, if you are married, it means terminating all flirtatious behavior with other women or men in the office. Maybe it means not going out to lunch alone with that colleague of the opposite sex.

ASSUME RESPONSIBILITY

The misuse of sex is not a private matter. God's design protects the goodness of committed relationships, either in the present or in the future. Except in the case of sexual abuse, if you have been sexually involved with someone who is not your spouse, you have in a way violated that person even though that person may have welcomed or even initiated the relationship.

More obviously, if you are married, any romantic extramarital liaisons are a violation of your spouse.

God expects us to ask others to forgive us when we have wronged them. This is especially important in the area of sexual sin, where emotions and hurt can run strong and deep. If you are single and dating, you might go to your girlfriend or boyfriend and say, "You know, last night I not only sinned against God, I wronged you as well. I have confessed that to God and he has forgiven me. Now, I'm asking for your forgiveness." When you make that kind of declaration, you reflect God's strength of character. It is one of the most powerful things you can do, even if your former partner does not see the relationship as wrong.

The point here is not to preach, and you don't need to expect much of a response. (Remember, the basis of your forgiveness comes from God, not from the other person.) But your words can serve to clear the air. Also, if the other person does not agree with your understanding that your former involvement was wrong, this meeting, even if it involves the exchange of forgiveness, should *not* be the basis for reactivating the relationship.

If you are married, it might be wise to seek the help of a Christian counselor or pastor before you ask your spouse's forgiveness. (Be sure to select a helper who acknowledges the wisdom of seeking forgiveness and is skilled in assisting reconciliation.) Do not underestimate the depth of hurt your behavior may have caused, and do not think everything will be cleared up in one brief conversation.

Here are a few practical guidelines for asking forgiveness.

- *Do not project blame on the other person.* For example, don't begin with, "I guess I need to ask you to forgive me, but it wasn't all my fault ..." or "If I was wrong ..." Such comments are just a backhanded way of blaming the other person. The other person may share responsibility for the situation. But you must deal with your part cleanly and completely first. Then, as part of the process of understanding or reconciliation, it might be appropriate for you to explain how the other person contributed.
- *Speak personally.* One young man could not face his girlfriend, so he asked her

forgiveness on videotape. The girl, a student at the time, was so offended by him that she played the tape through the school television system during lunch period! Don't document sin; God forgets it. We don't need a permanent record that could come back to haunt us later. Ask by phone or in person.

- *Don't be surprised if the other person won't forgive you.* Sometimes the only way a person can deal with his *own* guilt is to blame you. If he or she forgives you, that can upset the balance by removing his or her source of blame.

AVOID TEMPTATION

George's problem "began" when he was tempted to turn in to an X-rated theater on the way home from work. Two or three times a week he just couldn't resist. And sometimes when he came out, his next stop was a hot singles' bar, then the bedroom of the first girl he could pick up.

After these episodes, he felt great guilt but couldn't seem to break the cycle. He agreed that it was wrong. He would confess his sin and seek God's forgiveness. But nothing seemed to help. Then one day, when George was seeking the help of his pastor, his pastor asked which theater he found so irresistible. George told him, and the pastor thought a moment. "But George, isn't that theater four or five blocks out of your way when you walk home from work?"

Indeed it was. The theater marquee wasn't so irresistible; George had been making his decision about what was going to happen to him when he took the indirect route from work.

For George, fruit in line with repentance meant going straight home from work. And it became the first step in breaking his pattern of sexual misuse.

Avoiding temptation is critical if you want to experience the new start that can follow your clean heart. To restore "spiritual virginity," you must take away the avenue or environment for sin. You need to make a full about-face or the temptation to return can overwhelm you into reverting back to your old life-style. Saint Paul warned us to "make no provision for the flesh in regards to its lusts" (Romans 13:14, NASB). Hang in there with your convictions and you'll keep moving forward.

Joseph's determination to flee temptation shows the importance of this action. This man, described in the Bible in Genesis, was one of the leading patriarchs of Israel. When Joseph was the servant of Potiphar, a wealthy Egyptian nobleman, he had the responsibility of taking care of Potiphar's estate. Potiphar's wife was attracted to Joseph, and when Potiphar was away, she tried to seduce Joseph. She gave him every opportunity. In fact, she even begged him to go to bed with her. But he played it smart; he told her he could never sin against God and he got out of there.

She didn't give up. She finally caught him *alone*, grabbed his clothes, and wanted to make love. But Joseph didn't stay around and try to explain so he wouldn't hurt her feelings. He just split in a hurry.

The immediate consequence was far from positive. Potiphar's wife, angry at having been rejected, accused *Joseph* of being the one who made the advances. Framed in this way, Joseph was put in jail. But God delivered him from jail and raised him up to be one of the most powerful men in the world, second only to Pharaoh.

ESTABLISH ACCOUNTABILITY
Fruit in line with repentance might also mean saying to God that you're going to find someone to be accountable to. God encourages us to have a close friend who will help and encourage us in our relationship with Christ and in personal purity. "Two are better than one, because they have a good return for their work: If one falls down, his friend can help him up. But pity the man who falls and has no one to help him up!" (Ecclesiastes 4:9-10). As the apostle Paul added, we are to "encourage one another and build up one another" (1 Thessalonians 5:11, NASB).

If you're a woman, you may want to find a close girlfriend who shares God's standards, one who also wants her life to be pure. Go to that person and say, "Let's hold each other accountable in our moral lives." Begin to pray together for each other. If one is taking off for a party, the other can pray that she will stick to her standards.

Don't establish this accountability relationship with someone of the opposite sex. Praying together and discussing your feelings can be a very intimate experience. You could be asking for trouble. (Of course, if you have a struggle with homosexual attraction, don't set up a one-on-one relationship with the same-sex person. Possibly a group of three where at least one person has no homosexual inclination would work.)

In fact, I caution unmarried couples not to spend *a lot* of time together studying the Bible and praying alone. When you put a man and a woman in a very intimate spiritual relationship, the progression of the friendship can move quickly to the physical. You can end up in a physical relationship without even realizing it. That's why in marriage the closer you draw spiritually to your husband or wife, usually the greater your sex life becomes. It's uncanny! But true.

That doesn't mean you don't pray together. But when you do pray together, you should (1) make it very brief, (2) commit the time to the Lord, (3) pray for others, and, (4) pray positively. Don't pray about your loneliness or how you wish you didn't have to wait for sex until marriage. Those kinds of prayers are invitations to sexual intimacy. Your feelings (your loneliness and struggles) are legitimate, but they are best shared with close friends with whom you're not romantically involved.

EXPECT TESTING

Expect that any standards you set up will be tested. You will be tempted to pull back into a life-style that will create a wall between you and God.

Stand strong and be honest with the person to whom you are accountable. The only time you lose is when you quit or lower your standard. Realize that you have God rooting for you and that you can walk pure, even if your first steps are a little rough and shaky.

Bring forth fruit in line with repentance. And if it's an immoral relationship, and it looks like it might happen again, then you should break it off. What might feel like the end temporarily is really the beginning of something more wonderful than anything that you have left behind.

IT'S NEVER TOO LATE

The enemy of God, Satan, may try to make you feel guilty and hopeless even after you have accepted God's forgiveness. You may be plagued by feelings of remorse and worthlessness, feelings that keep you from God and the peace he offers you.

But Satan has no power over you! None! He'll work overtime, but he needn't succeed. Just stand firm and say right out loud, "I'm pure, I'm cleansed, and I'm a child of God with a personal relationship with Jesus Christ." Grab hold of Romans 8:28, where Saint Paul says, "And we know that God causes all things to work together for the good to those who love God, to those who are called according to his purpose."

Notice the above verse does not say all things are good. But, rather, that God will cause all things to *work together* for the good. Premarital or extramarital sex isn't good, but when we confess it and forsake it, God through His love and compassion can use it for your good. Don't let false guilt, prompted by Satan, get you down. Realize God loves you and that it's never too late to change.

One young woman came up to me at a student conference. She said, "Josh, I became a Christian two years ago, and some of the things that I did the first year as a Christian were dishonoring to God, to others, and to myself. I've confessed them to God and He has forgiven me, and now I am a walking example of how God can cause all things to work together for good. Almost every week, He has brought two or three girls into my path who are just at the point of becoming sexually involved, or who have just blown it, and they ask me what to do! And I am able to draw upon what I went through and then share my experience of God's grace and forgiveness to help them."

She was crying with *joy* as she explained how God had taken something that was bad in her life and is now using it for good and for His glory. It is never too late. Remember one thing: God is greater than any event in your life—past, present, and future.

RENEW YOUR MIND

To maintain your clean heart, it is important to do what the Bible calls renewing your mind. Saint Paul advises: "Therefore, I urge you, brothers, in view of God's mercy, to offer your bodies as living sacrifices, holy and pleasing to God—this is your spiritual act of worship. Do not conform any longer to the pattern of this world, but be transformed by the renewing of your mind. Then you will be able to test and approve what God's will is—his good, pleasing and perfect will" (Romans 12:1-2).

What is a renewed mind? A renewed mind is one that is totally reformed to be compatible with God's perspective.

One reason some people get this far, only to fall back into their old behavior, is that they are double-minded—that is, they have not fully made up their mind to exclusively pursue the singular path of sexual purity. Such a person has a split focus, one eye on what God wants and one eye on fleeting pleasures. Because he or she is not sold out to God 100 percent, every time a pressure comes along, he is moved in the direction of the pressure.

Renewal of your mind may need to begin with a little house cleaning. Men, how can you renew your mind and at the same time look at pornography? Some of you will have to throw out magazines or videotapes you have collected. You will never renew your mind and stay pure if you don't draw the line.

And women, some of you have popular women's magazines or romance novels that are not in tune with God's standards. Let's be honest. Some of you have used these magazines as your basis for defining love, and they've distorted your view.

FILL YOUR MIND WITH GOD'S WAYS
The process of renewing our minds is twofold. First, we do it through getting familiar with what God thinks by reading the Bible. The psalmist said, "How can a young man keep his way pure? By living according to your word. I seek you with all my heart; do not let me stray from your commands. I have hidden your word in my heart that I might not sin against you" (Psalm 119:9-11).

But we must do more than become knowledgeable. We must *think* God's

Word. Our goal should be to flush out the old thoughts we have stored in our minds and exchange them for God's thoughts.

Let's take it even a step farther. Suppose I meet you on the street and I ask you your name. You would respond without hesitation. You see, your name has become so familiar to you that it's part of your life. It literally is ingrained in your identity. God's Word must become that much a part of you.

This way, men, when you look at a woman on the beach, you don't think your former thoughts. They aren't controlled any longer by lust and fantasy. Instead, you think pure thoughts, such as, *God created women beautiful. . . that woman is the object of God's affection and may already be (or soon may become) the wife of someone else.*

IMMERSE YOURSELF
IN GODLY FRIENDSHIPS

Another way we can renew our minds is through friendships with people who model Christ-like world views. More and more, I am convinced that having friends who love Christ strengthens your convictions. Their relationship with God rubs off on you and vice versa. This is why Paul says, "Finally, brothers, whatever is true, whatever is noble, whatever is right, whatever is pure, whatever is lovely, whatever is admirable—if anything is excellent or praiseworthy—think about such things"

(Philippians 4:8). Why immerse ourselves in these things? Because they come from God, and when we think on them and surround ourselves with others who encourage the same, our attitudes and minds are changed.

We can thank God for making us sexual beings and for caring about us and our families and our love life. We can thank Him for giving us the strength to control our sexual desires.

DON'T FOCUS ON THE NEGATIVE

When old thought patterns come back to mind, acknowledge them; don't suppress them. In fact, acknowledge your sexuality; don't suppress it. Thank God that he created you a sexual being, with the desire and ability to have sex. Thank Him. Then acknowledge that He gave sex to be expressed within the context of a *loving* commitment of man and woman in marriage. Acknowledge that lust for premarital or extramarital expressions of sex is not in God's plan.

Don't say to yourself, *I'm not going to think about it . . . I'm not going to think about it.* Why? Because in fixating on resistance you are actually thinking about what you don't want to do!

Acknowledge that certain past acts or thoughts are sinful, then acknowledge that Christ died for them, that you've confessed them, and that you're forgiven. Each time you do this, you'll become stronger and more aware of God's forgiveness. Every time the thoughts come back, refocus your mind on Christ and His death for you on the cross. Saint Paul encouraged this when he wrote: "Set your mind on the things above" (Colossians 3:1, NASB).

Remember, no sin is too great for God to deal with. He wants to help. He loves you. He offers forgiveness and a new start with a clean heart. When He says, "clean," He means *clean!* And when He says "new," He means *new!* Your slate's clean and the sky's the limit. He never meant it any other way.

Dealing with Sexual Abuse

It was the most horrifying experience of my life . . .

I didn't want my "boyfriend" to do it . . . In fact, I told him no, but it didn't do any good. He did it to me anyway . . .

I was young and innocent . . . I didn't know what was really going on . . . I just knew that what my uncle was doing to me wasn't quite right . . .

I feel confused, guilty, dirty, and afraid to say anything about it to anyone . . .

If you have experienced some type of sexual abuse or think you have, you could be struggling with some pretty tough feelings: buried anger, hurt, guilt, or fear. You may or may not have been hurt physically, but deep inside you are probably suffering from some serious wounds. Just as a cut or a bruise needs treatment and time to heal, so does the hurt from sexual abuse. In time and with the proper treatment, many people who have been sexually abused have experienced emotional healing. You can, too.

A young woman wrote me recently and asked a question many who have been sexually abused have asked.

Dear Mr. McDowell,

When I was thirteen years old, my brother raped me. I am now nineteen and live on my own. What he did to me has left a very painful and emotional scar on my life which haunts me to this day.

I know I am not to blame for what happened to me, but why do I feel so guilty? Many times I feel like crawling inside a hole and never coming out. I don't want to feel so empty inside any more. I can't get back what I lost, but can I be forgiven for something that wasn't my fault?

—Raped at Thirteen

Why does this young lady feel guilty for something that wasn't her fault? She is not to blame for being raped; her offender is the one who is guilty. So why should she feel guilt?

Professional counselors tell us that even a small child can sense that sexual abuse is wrong. Children feel uncomfortable knowing that what's happening is somehow not right. That's because sex is out of its proper context—sex has been misused.

Adolescents, also, do not distinguish whose fault it is; they simply feel a violation has occurred. They have been made party to a delinquency and have engaged in the misuse of sex. The fact that it wasn't their choosing, even if they found it momentarily pleasurable, is not at issue. Their emotions simply feel wrong was done, leading them to accept guilt they don't actually own. A sexually abused person needs to realize that feelings of guilt occur because wrong was done, but *she or he is not the guilty party!*

Knowing and accepting we are not at fault does not automatically erase our feelings. But in time, as we accept that Christ died for all our sins, our emotions can be cleansed from the negative effects of wrongs forced on us. (See appendix 1 for more information from counselor Jan Frank.)

YOU'RE NOT ALONE

One of the most tightly guarded secrets in many people's lives is a history of sexual abuse. In the United States alone, one of every three women and one in six men have experienced at least one incident of sexual abuse before they turned eighteen! More than half of them will not tell anyone within a year of the assault. Do you know why? Most of them feel guilty and end up covering up the sexual abuse. Yet that generally makes it worse.

The one who has been abused needn't feel guilty because he or she is *the victim!* If you've been sexually abused, it's not your fault—you didn't cause it. You may have cooperated in some way or even been sexually aroused, but you're not the one responsible—it's not your fault!

Remember, victims are *never* responsible for or the cause of sexual abuse. So while it may be difficult and you may struggle with guilt, it is usually best to tell someone about the abuse rather than try to keep it a secret.

WHAT EXACTLY IS SEXUAL ABUSE?

Sexual abuse comes in many forms. It could be indecent exposure, obscene phone calls, Peeping Toms, the use of any kind of pressure or threats to force someone to participate in genital or oral stimulation, fondling, or sexual intercourse.

Of course, sexual abuse includes sexually violent acts such as rape, sadism, or any other type of physical abuse with sexual overtones.

Another form of abuse, incest, is sexual relations of any kind with a family member to whom one is not married—an uncle or aunt, a brother or sister, a stepbrother or stepsister, a mother or father, a grandparent, a stepparent, etc.

About 41 percent of the abusers in the United States are friends or acquaintances (i.e., date rape), 27 percent are strangers, and 23 percent are relatives (incest). In fact, nearly 75 percent of all rape and sexual assaults are done by people known to the victims.

Sexual abuse of any kind will usually not stop by itself. Rapists typically continue raping women until they are caught and imprisoned or given effective treatment. Incest or other sexual abuse in families usually continues until help from outside the family is secured. A guy who will date-rape a girl once will do it again unless there is some intervention.

If you are a victim of any form of sexual abuse, never rely on an offender's promise that it will never happen again as a reason to keep the incident a secret. Tell someone, and get help! Without outside help, the occurrences and the effects of the abuse are likely to go on for years or for life. Family relationships may become strained and painful. Anxiety and fear of closeness may get worse, and some victims act their feelings out in various ways such as becoming chemically dependent on alcohol or drugs. Eating disorders can also be a consequence. (Victims may subconsciously reason that if they get fat and therefore unattractive, the abuse will stop.)

Covering up sexual abuse usually makes its effects worse and can allow the effects to continue longer.

RAPE OR "DATE RAPE"

Rape is when sexual intercourse or oral sex is forced on you against your will. This could be by someone you know or by a complete stranger.

Rape is a violent crime and is against the law.

You may fear that people will think you're guilty or that you brought it on by the way you acted or dressed. The fact is that there is *never* an excuse for rape. Raping someone is *never* okay. The victim is *never* at fault. You do not cause someone else to commit a crime against you. Rape is something the offender chooses to do, and it is in no way your fault. You do not control another person's decision to violate you.

Date rape is when intercourse or oral sex is forced on you by the person you are dating. The "force" does not have to involve a weapon or even the threat of physical harm. It can involve trying to physically overpower a victim. But it can also involve intimidating threats like, "Hey, if you don't want to put out, you can get out of the car right now and walk home."

Rape or date rape is a violent crime and it's against the law. Yet you've probably heard some people say, "They brought it on themselves by the way they acted or dressed."

That's crazy!

Nobody has the right to rape another person, no matter what they've done! If someone forces sex on you, you're the victim and they're the law breaker. Remember, forced sex is not love; it's against the law!

SPEAK UP!
Because sexually abusing someone is against the law, speak up! Decide to tell someone the truth about what happened—a trusted friend, your pastor, a counselor, a doctor. The person you tell is required in most states to tell the local authorities. That's because all of us want sexual abuse to stop. And what about you—the victim? You need to be protected so it won't happen again.

And think of this: telling the truth may help stop the person from abusing you again or someone else. Telling can also be a help to you. One abuse victim said, "It is such a relief to know I don't have to hide any part of my life and to know that people accept me for what I am."

But telling isn't easy, either. What if some people won't believe you? If the abuser is someone you care about, it can get pretty confusing. You could be feeling anger and resentment toward the person and yet have some good memories and even love for them. It takes a lot of courage to speak out.

Many churches and communities have specialists in the area of sexual abuse and rape. Ask your school counselor, doctor, teacher, pastor, one of your friends' parents, or one of your own parents to help you locate help in your community.

WHAT YOU CAN DO TO AVOID DATE RAPE OR SEXUAL ABUSE

If you are in a situation where you have been sexually abused, there are a number of practical steps you can take to secure your safety. And that should be your first objective.

1. Try to avoid being alone with the abuser or anyone who wants to touch you in a sexual way. If you are uncomfortable around someone—maybe you feel fear about something and you don't even know why—trust your instincts. Avoid being alone with that person.

2. Don't deny that the abuse hurts you and you are angry about it. Talk to a trusted friend about the way you are feeling. Your feelings are not abnormal or weird; they are very normal.

3. Be reassured that sexual pressure of any kind is wrong. You never owe sexual favors to anyone no matter what the other person has done for you.

4. Set an example of how to treat guys and girls by mutually respecting each other. Sexual pressure of any kind is wrong.

5. Date only persons you know. Blind dates are always risky simply because you don't know the other person. Become friends before you go out alone on a date

with someone. Not only will you get to know something about the person's character, but your date will come to know you more as a person and not just a sex object.

6. Group dates with more than one couple could be helpful. An abuser or rapist usually needs to isolate his victim.

7. Don't go "parking." Avoid isolated situations or places.

8. Don't go into each other's home alone.

9. Respect others. Talking about or looking at another person in a way that makes them uncomfortable is not cool—it violates a person's dignity. Don't join in with friends who violate— verbally or physically—another person's space.

10. Believe that when someone says no to sex, she (or he) means no! Honor their feelings.

FACING YOUR FEELINGS

The emotional effects of sexual abuse can be very long lasting. Sometimes they are disguised in other symptoms. If you were abused in your past, you might ask yourself the following questions:

• Do you often feel hopeless, alone, and believe you are a burden to others?
• Do you find yourself withdrawing from family and friends?
• Do you have trouble concentrating?

If You've Been Sexually Abused

1. It was not your fault. It was a criminal act against you.
2. God does not condemn you. You are not "spoiled" or "dirty" in God's eyes.
3. The effects of abuse may influence your relationships over a long period of time. But you can recognize when this is happening and learn what you can do about it. You can recover. There is healing for you.
4. Reach out to trusted friends. Call them on the phone and tell them you need to talk or go see them.
5. Reach out to God. Talk to Him as you would your best friend. He is always there to listen and care. The Bible says, "Pour out your hearts to him,

• Do you have trouble excelling in your work or at school?
• Do you feel you have to keep "the secret"?

If you have been abused or raped and you answered yes to any of the preceding questions, you are normal. People who have experienced sexual abuse often have these feelings.

One abused person said, "I live in a dark, dark cavern of fear and isolation and guilt." You may feel very confused or fear that you won't be believed if you tell some-

70

for God is our refuge" (Psalm 62:8). "Cast all your anxiety on him because he cares for you" (1 Peter 5:7).

6. If the feelings get too tough to handle, start a journal by writing out how you feel at that moment. If you're afraid someone will read them, tear them up after you're finished or put them in a locked box.

7. There is hope—for you and also for the abuser. It is *never* too late to ask for help. God promises to heal wounds. One special promise can be found in 1 Peter 5:10: "The God of all grace, who called you to his eternal glory in Christ, after you have suffered a little while, will himself restore you and make you strong, firm and steadfast."

one. If the abuser is someone you care about, you are probably having mixed and confusing feelings of anger, hate, resentment, as well as more positive feelings such as love, good memories, and hopeful promises. These feelings need to be acknowledged, talked through, and resolved.

Keeping these feelings bottled up inside may only make the problem worse. Anger is a normal reaction to a loss—whether it's a physical loss or an emotional loss. All sexual abuse victims feel anger and need to express it in healthy ways. You don't

Promises from God

- God can heal your hurts!
  "He *heals the brokenhearted*. He bandages their wounds" (Psalm 147:3, ICB).
- You are a delight to God!
  "Because *he delights in me*, he saved me" (Psalm 18:19, ICB).
- God is your protector!
  "*God is our protection* and our strength. He always helps in times of trouble" (Psalm 46:1, ICB).
  "The Lord is close to everyone who prays to him, to all who truly pray to him. . . . He listens when they cry, and he saves them" (Psalm 145:18, 19b, ICB).
- God chose you to be His child!
  ". . . *he chose us* before the world was made. In his love *he chose us*" (Ephesians 1:4, ICB).
  "You did not choose me, *I chose you*" (John 15:15, ICB).
- God loves you and has a wonderful plan for your life!
  ". . . I know what I have planned for you . . . *I have good plans for you*. I don't plan to hurt you. *I plan to give you hope and a good future*" (Jeremiah 29:11, ICB).
  "For *God loved the world so much* that he gave his only Son. God gave his Son so that whoever believes in him may not be lost, but have eternal life" (John 3:16, ICB; italics added here and above).

have to be angry all the time. You can begin to take charge of your life. You can learn to trust your own judgment and get close to others and yet remain in control. This process may take years, but there is hope for you. Pastors, counselors, your doctor, a support group, or trusted friends can provide much help as you struggle to get free from your past experiences.

Questions about Abuse

The following questions were put to Jan Frank, a licensed counselor, victim of sexual abuse, and author of the book A Door of Hope, *published in 1987 by Here's Life Publishers.*

Is sexual abuse a problem in our society today?

Yes, most definitely. Some of the current research indicates that about one out of every three women in the United States today has been sexually molested by the time she is eighteen years of age. The statistic for men is about one out of six.

Why look at something that happened a long time ago? Doesn't the Scripture say that we are to "forget those things that are behind" and press forward?

Yes, the Scripture does say that. However, as we look at the context of that passage in Philippians 3, we see that in the preceding verses Paul actually recounts his past. The emphasis of verse 13 is that we not dwell or wallow in the past in such a way as to prevent us from moving toward the goals that God has for us. I have found in working with many people that a failure to look into one's past may result in actually carrying out some very destructive patterns in adult life.

When we have been sexually abused, there are some coping mechanisms we learn to help us survive a hurtful situation. These may include compulsive behaviors like overeating, becoming an overachiever, or compulsively exercising. When a child has been abused, he receives messages about himself, about others, and about God that are very distorted. Unless these issues are addressed, a person grows into adulthood with a warped view of who he/she really is and who God is.

I believe that God is the one who is causing many of these issues to be addressed because He is grieved at the way we have been traumatized. He sees how every area of our life has been affected by these events: our inability to trust others; our lack of self-worth; our inability to give and receive love from others and from God; our distorted view of God; and our difficulty in living the abundant life. It is because of His great desire that we have an undistorted relationship with one an-other—and, more importantly, with Him—that He brings many of these hurtful events to the surface, because they have a way of robbing us from the very relation-ship that He so longs to have with us.

If young people don't address these issues now, what is likely to occur?
For me, the most significant impact oc-curred in the area of my relationships. As a young person, I found myself attracted to people who were not healthy for me. Even though I was a Christian, I seemed to get into dating relationships with young men who were emotionally abusive or emotion-ally dependent.

Due to unresolved issues in our back-ground, we are often magnetized to others who have come from dysfunctional homes. The problem with this is that it becomes a cycle carried from generation to genera-tion (see Exodus 34:6-7). Unless we recog-nize, root up, and resolve these issues, we will be prone to reproduce the dysfunction when we marry and have families.

As I have worked with many couples, I have seen what a very tragic effect has resulted when abuse has not been dealt with adequately in the beginning. Even in my own relationship with my hus-band, Don, who is a wonderful Christian man, we have observed many destructive patterns that we both brought into our marriage due to some unresolved family-of-origin issues.

These issues do not go away. There was a woman in my first support group who was sixty-six years old. She confessed she had carried the secret of what had happened to her and all the anger, betrayal, and confusion for over fifty years. Unfortunately, most people try to bury it, only to find out that the memories, emotions, and trauma resurrect themselves later on in life.

Is it possible for someone who has been sexually abused to have no ill effects?
No, I do not believe so. Most victims struggle with being able to trust others. They often feel guilty or ashamed for what has happened. They may feel dirty, bad, or used. They commonly have a poor self-image and have trouble being able to fully grasp and accept God's love for them.

Some of the consequences of the abuse may mask themselves until later in life. I became an overachiever in high school and college, desperately trying to compensate for the deep insecurity and inadequacy I felt inside.

Most people saw me as a confident, hard-working perfectionist who was compulsively driven to excel. They did not see my struggle with rejection, my intense need for control, or the battle I went through to believe from my heart that God really did love me.

What are the signs and symptoms that result when someone has been sexually abused?
I have already mentioned a few, but let me list some other symptoms that can indicate major, unresolved hurts:

- Chronic depression (feeling down on a regular basis)
- Displaced anger (excessive anger over other minor causes)
- Fears or phobias
- Panic attacks
- Eating disorders such as compulsive overeating, bulimia (binge eating and purging), anorexia (self-starvation)
- Unfounded shame or guilt
- Lapses of memory of childhood (gaps of time that are missing)
- Difficulty in establishing relationships or poor choices in relationships
- Lesbian or homosexual tendencies
- Promiscuity
- Compulsive masturbation
- Drug abuse
- Migraine headaches
- Stomach problems

There are several other sources for any of these symptoms, so one should not jump to conclusions—particularly in "diagnosing" someone else. But if you have a history of having been abused sexually and are struggling with some of these symptoms without other satisfactory explanations, the abuse may be the source.

If a person recognizes some of these symptoms in his or her life, what steps should be taken?

First, a person needs to begin to pray and ask God for direction. Some victims feel that these issues can be resolved between themselves and God alone. God is able to heal us totally without any assistance from another human being. However, He often uses people in the healing process to minister to us directly.

I encourage victims to seek professional, Christian counseling with someone who understands the problems of the sexually abused. If such a person is not available, a person needs to find knowledgeable support persons who have educated themselves through reading books or attending seminars on victimization and who have an understanding of the issues that need to be addressed.

Part of the trauma the child feels when she has been abused is that she goes through the experience alone. An integral part of the healing is walking through the pain of what happened with a loving, supportive person who embodies the unconditional love of God.

If you go to someone who says, "Just forget it and go on with your life," recognize that this person may be well-meaning but does not understand that these issues do not disappear by pretending they are not there. Don't quit! Search until you find a counselor, pastor, or mature Christian who is willing to walk alongside you in your journey toward wholeness in God.

How do you know if you've gotten over it?
Very simply, the symptoms will begin to disappear. After I went into counseling and worked through some of the rage, bitterness, and anger I had buried inside for so many years, I saw a dramatic decrease in my migraine headaches. I found I was able to begin to trust my husband and establish healthy relationships with others.

I caution people regarding "quick recovery." Almost every letter I receive in the mail tells a woman's story of her victimization—what she is currently struggling with. But invariably it concludes with, "But I know I've resolved these issues because I've forgiven my abuser." If a person continues to carry with them a majority of the symptoms I described earlier, it often means they have *not* dealt fully enough with some of the deeper roots.

The healing of an abusive past is a developmental issue. That means that it goes in stages. What I could not deal with as a single adult at twenty, I may be equipped to deal with at twenty-seven. What I am dealing with at thirty-five is different from what God will bring up at forty-five. Life and healing is a process.

The Scripture tells us that we are in the process of "being conformed to the image of His Son" (see Romans 8:29), but that we can be "confident of this very thing, that He will complete the work that He has begun in us" (see Philippians 1:6).

I am healed. But I am also in the process of being healed. God has completed that work in the Spirit, but it takes time to accomplish in the flesh that which is already accomplished in the Spirit.

What are the steps toward healing?
The steps God took me through for healing are outlined and detailed in my book, *A Door of Hope.* Briefly, these are the steps God took me through. They form the acronym "Free to Care."

F-ace the problem
R-ecount the incident
E-xperience the feelings
E-stablish responsibility

T-race behavior difficulties/symptoms
O-bserve others and educate yourself

C-onfront the aggressor
A-cknowledge forgiveness
R-ebuild self-image and relationships
E-xpress concern and empathize with
others

I share in my book that these are not ten easy steps that you can decide to do over the next two months or even six months. God deals with us individually. But these steps can be used as a guideline to some of the issues that need to be addressed.

Please note: The step of confrontation is *not* appropriate for a child or adolescent. In fact, confrontation is not always appropriate for a young adult. If it is to take place, it must be done as an adult after much prayer and under the consultation of a professional.

Can someone ever get over the pain that has resulted from these events?
Absolutely. It may take time, but God desires that we live abundantly in Him. He wants us to live in fullness of joy in our relationship with Him. He knows unresolved abuse issues are blockages or obstacles in our relationship with Him, so it is His Spirit that "leads us into all truth" (see John 16:13). We are told that we "shall know the truth and the truth shall set us free" (see John 8:32).

If I deal with these issues as a single person, is it necessary for me to tell my mate about it when I marry?
Yes. No matter how much one tries to deal with these issues as a single person, residue will likely arise when you marry, particularly in the sexual area. I believe during premarital counseling this topic should be addressed. I was not able to go into a lot of detail with my husband, Don, about what happened before we were married. However, I did share that I had been sexually

abused. Don did not understand all the ramifications of those events in my life, but I am certainly glad that I told him.

I believe there needs to be a great deal of prayer and forethought about sharing the details of our past with our potential mate. I often encourage couples to seek counseling from a pastor, a well-known friend, or someone whose marriage you respect to seek counsel on these sensitive issues.

Where was God when all this happened?
This was a question I asked in the midst of my own recovery. I encourage victims to be honest with God about their feelings and to ask Him some of those very tough questions. He spoke to me very personally through His Word when I asked Him this question, and I am sure that He will speak to you, too.

God never calls evil good. He was not the one who orchestrated the abuse in my life. It is because of human sinfulness that these tragic events occur. It is also because Satan desires to "steal and kill and destroy" (John 10:10). I believe it was Satan's plan that these events take place, not only to destroy me but to destroy my family as well. Praise God that He is a God of redemption and healing. He promises us that He "will restore the years the locusts have eaten" (see Joel 2:25), and He has truly done that in my life.

He is able to redeem anything when we yield it into His loving hands.

One of my favorite verses in Scripture is Isaiah 49:15-16 (AMP), which says: "Can a woman forget her nursing child, that she should not have compassion on the son of her womb? Yes, they may forget, yet will I not forget you. Behold, I have indelibly imprinted (tattooed) a *picture* of you on the palm of each of My hands."

I know that God never lost sight of that ten-year-old child who was wounded so long ago. He loved me then, as He loves me now, and He has taken the "valley of trouble" in my life and made it a "door of hope."

Jesus came to "bind up the broken-hearted and to set at liberty the captives" (see Luke 4:18). He wants to do that in our lives. God promised in Ezekiel 36:34-36:

> The desolate land will be cultivated instead of lying desolate in the sight of all who pass through it. They will say, "This land that was laid waste has become like the garden of Eden; the cities that were lying in ruins, desolate and destroyed, are now fortified and inhabited." Then the nations around you that remain will know that I the LORD have rebuilt what was destroyed and have replanted what was desolate. I the LORD have spoken, and I will do it.

APPENDIX
2

Resources You Can Use

Botkin-Maher, Jennifer. *Nice Girls Don't Get Raped* (San Bernardino, Calif.: Here's Life, 1987).

Didato, Victoria Kepler. *One in Four* (Mansfield, Ohio: Social Interest Press, 1984).

Frank, Jan. *A Door of Hope*, (San Bernardino, Calif.: Here's Life, 1987)

McDowell, Josh. *Building Your Self-Image* (Wheaton, Ill.: Tyndale, 1984).

——. *Love, Dad* (Waco, Tex.: Word, 1988).

——. *The Secret of Loving* (Wheaton, Ill.: Tyndale, 1985).

McDowell, Josh, and Paul Lewis . *Givers, Takers, and Other Kinds of Lovers* (Wheaton, Ill.: Tyndale, 1980).

Purnell, Dick. *Free to Love Again: Coming to Terms with Sexual Regret* (San Bernardino, Calif.: Here's Life, 1989).

What Everyone Should Know About the Sexual Abuse of Children, A Scriptographic Booklet by Channing L. Bete Co., Inc., South Deerfield, Mass., 1987.

About the Author

JOSH McDOWELL is one of the most popular speakers on the world scene today. In the last twenty-three years he has given more than 18,000 talks to over 8 million students and faculty at 1,000 universities and high schools in seventy-two countries. Josh is author of thirty-two best-selling books and has been featured in twenty-seven films and videos and two TV specials.

Josh graduated cum laude from Kellogg College in economics and business. He finished graduate school magna cum laude with degrees in languages and theology. He is a member of two national honor societies and was selected by the Jaycees in 1976 as one of the "Outstanding Young Men in America." He holds honorary doctorate degrees in law and theology.

Josh and his wife, Dottie, have four children and live in Julian, California.

Let's Stay In Touch!

If you have grown personally as a result of this material, we should stay in touch. You will want to continue in your Christian growth, and to help your faith become even stronger, our team is constantly developing new materials.

We are now publishing a monthly newsletter which will:

1 tell you about those new materials as they become available
2 answer your tough questions
3 give creative tips on being an effective parent
4 let you know our ministry needs
5 keep you up to date on my speading schedule (so you can pray).

If you would like to receive this publication, simply fill out the coupon below and send it in. By special arrangement our newsletter will come to you regularly--no charge.

Let's keep in touch! *Josh*

Yes Josh! *I want to receive the free subscription to your newsletter.*

Name_____

Address_____

City_____State_____Zip_____

Mail to: Josh McDowell • Campus Crusade for Christ
           Arrowhead Springs • San Bernardino, CA 92414

SLC-2024

Why believe in Jesus Christ?

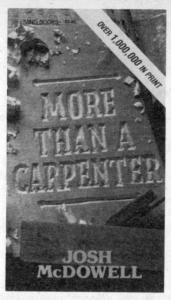

POCKET GUIDES
ALSO FROM TYNDALE

Christianity: Hoax or History? by Josh McDowell. Was Jesus Christ a liar, a lunatic, or Lord? A popular speaker and author looks at the resurrection of Jesus and other claims of the Christian faith. 72-0367-7 $2.95.

Hi-Fidelity Marriage by J. Allan Petersen. A respected family counselor shows you how to start an affair--with your spouse. Learn how to keep love alive...rekindle old flames...grow from mistakes. 72-1396-6 $1.95.

How to Talk to Your Mate by H. Norman Wright. Here are key elements to loving communication in marriage. Learn how to cope with conflict, handle fear and anger, and encourage each other. 72-1378-8 $2.95.

Surefire Ways to Beat Stress by Don Osgood. A thought-provoking plan to help rid your life of unhealthy stress. Now you can tackle stress at its source--and win. 72-6693-8 $2.25.

Five Steps to a Perfect Wedding by Ruth Muzzy and R. Kent Hughes. Take the hassle out of your wedding plans. This convenient guide helps you organize your rehearsal dinner, ceremony, and reception. Practical advice lets you know your options before you chose. 72-0899-7 $1.95.

POCKET GUIDES